Nutrition:

The Ultimate Beginners' Guide For Nutrition and Good Health

Introduction

I want to thank you and congratulate you for downloading the book, *"Nutrition: The Ultimate Beginners' Guide For Nutrition and Good Health.*

This book contains proven steps and strategies on how to have achieved nutritional balance.

We did our research and asked the experts. Because we didn't want to get sued by the big wigs in the nutrition industry, we left out some of the names. We did get some information from some major nutritional experts. We'll let you guess who we wrote about. This is an insider's guide. We have the insight, we did the research — we don't want to get sued.

Thanks again for downloading this book, I hope you enjoy it!

Chapter 1

Getting Started: The Ins and Outs of Food Addiction

Like other addictions, food addiction will make a person simply seek out their drug of choice and find excuses to keep the addiction going. One example is pushing away of family members who don't follow the same life guidelines as them. As a child of food addicts, I watched them say things to my daughter while they were dealing with type II diabetes. I'll always remember one parent say to my daughter, "Did you get your little tummy full?"

I got my daughter away from that as fast I could. See, food addiction is one of the most complicated addictions. It's not like alcohol or drugs. An addict can get away from that stuff. You can't do that with food. Good, simple food really is essential. Our bodies need food to live. You can get way from drugs, you can't get away from food. It is a necessity of life. If you don't do it right, you could end up nutritionally deprived.

I know you're asking right now, why you should listen to someone like me. Well, I was raised on a farm, I was raised in a blue zone and the only reason I escaped the food addicts was because I have a chronic illness that causes me to not like food. I eat for nutritional purposes. I've taught nutrition and I've done post-bachelor work in nutrition and I'm now studying nutrition and hope to one day hold a PhD in it.

I've seen the gleam in a food addict's eye and seen the anger emitted from them when they didn't get the food they craved.

I'll always remember one of the food addicts give my daughter an Easter basket and at the last minute take a nibble off an ear of a chocolate bunny. They saw and they took.

See, we are programmed to do this. We need food to thrive. Once food becomes more than a simple nourishment, it lands in the world of addiction.

Food should be enjoyed. It's been a part of human culture for centuries, and is part of togetherness. So what's the difference? How can food be a comfort an an addiction. Well, I'm not an addiction expert. I recently asked a counselor about arachnophobia or fear of spiders.

I simply didn't understand how a person could be scared of spiders. Well, it is a genuine worry. It's caused from learning from people in your environment. A person learns this by seeing other people close to them scared of the same thing. Much like food addiction, arachnophobia is developed from seeing others with the same fear. That's how the culture of food addiction can really take hold. If you are raised in an environment you are more likely to adopt their same eating habits. Until recently, food wasn't as readily available as it is now. I remember sitting next to a PhD and asking her what will be the downfall of America. She simply said Type II Diabetes, because everyone is getting it and it costs a lot of money to control. See, it can be controlled through diet. I was once blind to how addicted to food my own family was. I remember how when one parent was in the hospital with diabetic neuropathy and I went into their house and exchanged foods with sugar to sugar-free. It didn't go well.

That's because I didn't realize that the connection to sugar was emotional.

I consider myself lucky in many ways to have not adopted their food patterns. I do, however, know that hereditary I am predisposed to being a food addict. This genuinely scares me.

That's why I've always loved my dirt more.

With dirt you can grow your own food. If you are someone who thinks you may be a food addict, instead of going on another diet consider just slowing down the way you get food. If you are preparing your own food, you will then slow down how much time you spend eating. When I lived with the food addicts, I gained a bunch of weight. I had candy bars at the ready and fast food wasn't just an option. It happened regularly. Instead of beating yourself up about nutrition, just cut out the fast food. If that's hard for you, cut it back. A little self control will go a long way.

I was diagnosed with a rare disorder that I have had my entire life. I had been going to the hospital Emergency Room for years and they knew me and labeled me a Frequent Flyer. I wasn't diagnosed until my daughter was two. She loved watching the nurses and medical staff use latex gloves to blow up balloons. I won't find out for years what that experience did to her. I do know that she got to see her mother slowly get better. Once I was diagnosed, I began studying nutrition and started exercising. I changed my diet and stopped going to the Emergency Room.

I am learning to live like I'm not dying. I effectively healed myself and learned to live with chronic illness. There was nothing doctors could do. I did it through nutrition. I've already taken nutrition and am working towards a PhD in nutrition.

This illness is the reason I am not a Food Addict. There isn't a food that I haven't regurgitated. In many ways I do have a lot to thank for having this illness. Watching Food Addicted family members cope blindly with their love of empty calories was an eye-opening experience. I will always carry those memories with me. Not only was it eye-opening, it really put into perspective how I want to live out the rest of my days. I don't want to die from cancer, diabetes or obesity.

I know that Food Addiction is both a genetic factor and a factor in the environment I was raised. That's why I am hoping to live a life with a diet based on plant sources.

We live in a world full of processed food. It's easy for someone to engage in eating empty calories and eating foods out of a box. My plan is to adopt a healthy diet in order to not die from cancer, diabetes or obesity. See, I have a mitochondrial disease and through nutrition I learned how to keep my mitochondria in top notch shape by eating healthy diet and engaging in exercise. Why I do recommend eating mostly plants I do think we all should eat meat. We do eat too much meat in this country. Meat should never be bigger than your fist and most of your plant should be filled with fruits and vegetables. The biggest killer in the United States are preventable diseases. Most of these deaths could be prevented with a healthy diet.

Diabetes is a huge cause of early death. I'll always remember seeing a beloved family member inject her stomach every day with insulin. Not only was this medicine super expensive, it had to be refrigerated. That meant limiting her movement as her medicine had to be accounted for.

I spent nearly two hours trying to convince her caregiver that she needed medical help. After finally doing so I found out she was having a blood sugar crash and would have died had I not intervened when I did. An acquaintance of mine with a daughter with juvenile diabetes talked to me about her frustration with people with Type II Diabetes. "You can control your diabetes with diet with Type II. I have to watch my daughter.

What We Covered

- Food Addiction

- A Plant-Based Diet

- Disease Prevention

Chapter 2

Avoiding Heart Disease

Hundreds of thousands of people die from this disease. This is the number one killer of Americans. It doesn't need a pill or a vaccine. A fork will do. Fatty deposits in the arteries or the blood vessels that surround the heart causes a process that causes chest pain and can form a blood clot causing a heart attack. This is called Sudden Cardiac Death. Many people succumb to this and the first symptom is a lot of times your last. Many people assume this happens as you get older. It is not a necessary thing to deal with. It can be prevented. In places in China, no one even knows about coronary heart disease. This disease is preventable. A simple diet change will do it.

They have attributed this to the low cholesterol in the diet. These people eat lots of fiber and mainly a plant-based diet. Generations of people didn't get cavities until the invention of the candy bar.

Now that you're hating on the SAD diet or the American Standard Diet, let's talk about supplements. The first one we will talk about is fish oil supplements. They did a recent study where they found no benefit from them.

Heart Disease does start in childhood. Researchers did a study of people in 1993 and showed that Coronary Heart Disease were found in children by the age of ten. By the time we are 40 or 50 people start dying. It really isn't about prevention, it's also about reversal. These lesions start in childhood or even pregnancy.

To reduce your LDL levels, you need to eat less animal products and processed junk. Bad food really is an epidemic, not just a fad to be corrected. If you go to your physician today they are likely to give you a prescription for a medicine. Yes, these meds are important. If there is a fire going on, it must be extinguished before you really examine what caused the fire. However, eating a healthy diet can prevent any and all chronic illnesses. Take my chronic illness. It is connected to my mitochondria and once I changed by diet and started exercising, I stopped being sick all the time.

It changed my life.

The thing about baking, is that people do like to do it. They like to bake sweet goods and give them to others. They aren't thinking they are killing people with kindness.

There's a thing called the Tomato Effect. This refers to how the modern thought during one time was that tomatoes were bad for you. This was the consensus of the culture at the time. The same thing goes along with cigarettes. There was a time when it was said cigarettes were only bad for you in excess. Take everything in moderation.

When you hear the term Registered Dietician, you are hearing that a person is registered with an organization. Remember there was a time when doctor's used to recommend certain cigarettes.

Taking care of someone dying from obesity changed me. I will never be the same.

The way she denied her sugar habit. The way she always injected herself with insulin. How her quality of life was so diminished and her corpulent body prevented her from doing anything but sit on the couch and watch television. We all need to take care of our bodies.

Lung disease kills a huge amount of people per year. This too is preventable. It can in some ways be preventable with the inclusion of plants in your diet. Asthma is too preventable with avoidance of smoke and maintaining a healthy diet. It is said that with twenty minutes of quitting smoking your body begins to heal. The human body can heal itself. Yes cigarettes harm you and can harm your DNA. Foods like broccoli can heal your body. Cruciferous vegetables heal the body and can prevent damage. In a study from 2010 they found that cruciferous vegetables can prevent cancer cells from spreading. Turmeric is also said to help. It can prevent the initial DNA damage that occurs when you harm your body. Researchers have found that an ingredient in turmeric is a known stop of mutated DNA. Other plant-based foods do help the body. A typical meal should have a small protein and the rest of your plate should be mostly fruits and vegetables. Personally, I love vegetables so this isn't an issue. However, there are a lot of people who do not like vegetables. This stems from how you were fed as a baby. When you are beginning to feed a baby and introducing to them new foods, don't start with a bitter vegetable and don't start with a sweet fruit. Start with a vegetable that is bland. We recommend a squash.

Do an orange vegetable per week and then move on to green vegetables. Save the fruits for last. That initial shock when you introduce a baby a bitter vegetable first can cause a lifetime of vegetable hatred. Every time they see a vegetable they will have a flash back.

The consumption of cured meat can increase COPD. This is thought to be from the nitrates in meats like hot dogs. With a boost of the vegetable diet, the disease progression was halted. The antioxidants in the vegetables seemed to counteract the cured meat. That's how food works off each other. Meat does provide protein and at the same time cause harm. Vegetables do provide disease prevention and have phytochemicals. They are good for you.

Most Western diets are only recommended a small amount of fruits or vegetables. The simple act of adding more vegetables and fruits to your diet has halted diseases. Now you may be asking if you can just take a pill. Well, it doesn't seem to work this way. A whole-food diet rich in plants cannot be put into a pill. That's why eating whole-foods is paramount. Researchers in Sweden recently did a study of people with severe Asthma. More than 70-percent of patients got better by eating a whole foods diet.

It really can't hurt you. There is very little negative after-affects of eating a healthy diet. If you are someone who doesn't want to change the way you eat, consider taking small steps and do not guilt yourself if you fail. We are all hard enough on ourselves and if you don't eat right today, try again tomorrow. There is never a bad time to build a healthy diet habit.

• Plant-Based Dieting

• Whole-Food Diets

• Developing a Healthy Diet

• Quitting Smoking

Chapter 3

Diet Fads and Fiber: What does it all mean?

We all want a magic cure for our ailments.

All of us wish we could take a pill and live longer, not age and cure all our ailments. People have been selling snake oil since the dawn of humanity.

They've made money off the lie that is a magic remedy.

The truth is that life is pain. One of my favorite quotes is "Life is pain. Anyone who tells you different is selling you something." Please leave a review with the movie this quote comes from for a chance to win something.

There's no magic cure for illness. There is disease prevention and it comes from healty habits, not two-week magic remedies. Avoiding fast or convenient food can help, but that too is just suppressing the symptom. You should ask yourself what is going on in your mind that is causing you to crave comfort food? Yes, food does bring comfort. I remember when I worked as a social worker and one of my clients was crying. My instinct was to make her a plate of yummy food. I wanted to make her feel better and this was how I was taught to make someone feel better and even solve their problems.

Yes, marketing magicians may lead you to believe that if you eat a certain food you will be skinny. This is more pseudo-science than anything and is a form of snake oil. What matters is how many calories you put in versus what you burn. That's where diet and exercise play a huge factor.

Know that in life what you put in your mouth matters. It's not just how much you put down your gullet, it's what. There's this thing called empty calories. Those are processed foods such as French fries. Yes they are made from potatoes and deep fried thus making them delicious. You can take the same amount of fries and put them next to a baked potato and have the same calories and not the same nutrition. The processing of potatoes to fries takes out the nutrition. Potassium is a necessary ingredient in a potato. My clients who I coach and have the same disease as me are instructed to eat a potato a day. You could even say, "A potato a day will keep the deathbed away."

I say that because that is the number one way people with my chronic illness die. I remember one time I went to the Emergency Room and when they tested my blood they found that I had seriously low levels of potassium. A lot of the people who have died from my disease, died because their potassium levels crashed and they suffered a heart attack and died.

That is why I write about nutrition and continue to study it. See, when I was finally diagnosed I decided to go back to school and learn everything I could about the human body and try to find a cure. The thing is I found everything I needed to know in my nutrition class. I learned that certain vitamins aid the mitochondria and in cell production. Once I found my food trigger my life changed. I had renewed energy and joint pain went away. Stomach pain went away too. See, when I started on my Journey to Wellness, I had a hard time with fiber. I had to get back slowly. Believe it or not, fiber is important. It collects fatty deposits that you then poop out. It binds to things like cholesterol and gets them out of your system. Remember how I said take everything in moderation. No food is inherently bad for you. If you eat fast food do it sparingly. Just don't overdo it. Most nights of the week should be at home with a cooked meal. If all the adults in your family have jobs outside the home gadgets like instapots make making a wholesome meal easy. If there's a will, there's a way. You can make dinner for your family and make it wholesome too.

The easiest way to get fiber in your diet is by eating green-leafy vegetables. See, vegetables have this wonderful thing in them called phytochemicals. All scientists know is that they are important. They won't specify as to why. Personally, I think all whole food is necessary and it does work together to nourish and heal the body. Good nutrition is important and was one of the tenants of the philosephor behind the Hippocratic oath to do no harm. Doctors are healing However it is with pills not food.

Amazon is changing the way we shop. They have stores in big cities that you simply walk into and get what you want and it takes the money straight from your bank account. Not everyone wants to grow food, not everyone wants slow food.

It's about finding a guilt-free way to live your best food life.

If you are someone who believes the hype and tries the latest diet fad you will not find the magic road to good health. In order to do that you must monitor the calories that come in against what you burn. If you are hesitant to go visit the gym, think about taking a walk first. Ease your mind and relax into the wonderful world of diet and exercise. Eating healthy really is easy and it really is simple. It's about staying away from processed and fast food. If that is thought to be too difficult, start out small. Start with the easiest thing to cut out. So, it's easy to switch from a large soda to a small? Start with that. Things can change. Diets are variable.

Now look at you…

You are ready to start adding fiber and getting away from fad diets. Believe it or not, diseases like anorexia and bulimia are listed as nutritional disorders. These diseases happen when a person intentionally denies themselves nutrition. This does have side effects. Even people on the other side of anorexia can go back if they see a photo of a think woman. This is a trigger for this disease.

The best thing a person can do to prevent diseases like overeating and anorexia is to monitor their diet and choose a lifestyle that is active and full of whole food. That is why diseases like this are so difficult. One does not get away from food. It is about living a life of nutritional moderation. Yes, fast food does taste good. It's not an every day food. Yes, dessert tastes good. It's also not an everyday food. The American food pyramid is vastly different in this country compared to places around the world. Don't be xenophobic about your diet. Other countries recommend colorful vegetables and say that everyone should eat a variety of foods each day.

The easiest way to life a healthy lifestyle is to cook as much food as you can and eat as many vegetables as you can. Food should be enjoyed. It is not to be thought of as a punishment. It is not a reward system. Food is to be slow prepared and made wholesome for the entire family.

• What Is Fiber?

• The Food Pyramid.

• Anorexia and Bulimia

• Overeating

• Diet Fads

Chapter 4

All You Need is Fat and Calories

Let's start with omnivores and herbivores. I'll always remember sitting in my living room and watching a pigeon fly into my living room window and lay motionless on the ground. I went out to check on it and saw that the impact had killed him. I went back inside to get ready to remove the body and before I could grab my gear my chickens attacked. They circled the bird and devoured it before I had a chance to clean it up. See, chickens are said to be vegetarians. Well, yes and no. They will eat a bug and they will eat the recently deceased. That's why when you buy eggs laid from vegetarian hens that's either so true that the facility is completely closed and the hens are also caged, or it is a blatant lie. Your best bet is to find a local farm that sells eggs. The more natural the better. Many Farmers Markets sell eggs and other meat from their small farms.

The more whole foods you can buy the better. I'll also remember teaching young mothers about organic and they were raised to think of organic as bad. To them, organic meant more expensive and they were taught to avoid the organic label. I too think this is awful. Organic shouldn't be a food accesses only by those who can afford it. I also remember working at a school and watching the kids drink milk from plastic bags. All I could think about is the harmful chemicals leaching into their milk.

The slower the food and the closer to home you buy it the better. There is a thing called food deserts where local food is inaccessible. The people who live in these areas may not have access to buying local calories.

To ingest or not to ingest: that is the question you should ask. Everyone should have access to the nutrients needed to feed their bodies. That's why overeating is such a huge issue.

Early death brought on by overeating kills nearly as many people each year as tobacco. Track your BMI and if you are eating to much, don't remove the calories. Get moving and get making your food. When I graduated college I wanted to become a doctor. I couldn't handle the vomiting and didn't learn until much later I had a chronic illness and not a weak immune system. I treated my illness through vast study of nutrition.

Am I perfect: no. I know now how to put food into my body that heals it. Food really is medicine. Eat the wrong food and you could be harming and not helping your body. That's why my life is now dedicated to improving the nutrition in all aspects of life. Your health is directly connected to what you put in it. Are you eating fast food every day? You may want to cut that back. Eat another salad or take a walk. I've authored several books on the Ketogenic diet. It does fascinate me. I've seen a number of success stories from it. Like all diets, this one should be done in moderation.

For me, I eat a very Paleo diet. I avoid processed foods and eat rice. Because of my chronic illness I have to be careful what I put in my body. In my perspective my body is a temple and I am to honor it not destroy it. That's why I don't guilt myself if I fail one day. I simply pick myself up and try again be it at the gym or at the dinner table.

This morning I made treats with marshmallows. I don't plan on eating the entire tray. It really is about moderation. People selling you diet trends want you to feel bad about your diet. That is a marketing scheme to get you to buy their product. Don't fall for it. If anyone tries to tell you life isn't anything but hard work, they are trying to sell you something. Life is pain.

When you are looking at your nutrition labels, all you really need to know is don't eat anything you can't pronounce. Do everything you can to avoid added flavors or sugar. I remember going into a local grocer and trying their bread. It tasted good. Most breads are loaded with additives. Vegetables actually do taste good and ranch is a good thing to dip your carrots into. A combination of fat is needed to fully release the Vitamin A into your system. Fat isn't all bad.

If you were comparing a tiger to a cow who would you identify as fat? Know that tigers are meat eaters and cows eat mostly grass and grain. What makes them different? The amount of exercise they get. A tiger gets way more exercise and it really does show. Exercise does fit into a healthy diet. I found out through nutrition study that exercise does benefit the body.

I remember sitting next to a woman who did discuss the dangers of Type II Diabetes. I'll always remember that and accompany it with the study of how maintaining a proper weight can prevent disease. Proper nutrition can be done. If you are suffering with thinking of the culture or environment, know that it really is easy to make exceptions to your diet. It is okay to love someone and not love all they do. It is okay to occasionally indulge in desserts and fast food. Just don't let it become a habit. That's the nature of food addiction. We guilt ourselves and through that guilt we struggle and only think we can make our life better by loosing weight. This action feeds into the old adage of feeling fear and then buying something.

K now that only you can improve the nutrition you choose to ingest. It is solely your responsibility and if you fail it isn't someone else's fault. Living a life and changing your nutrition habits take time. If you fail, try again. We live in a world with food deserts and fast food joints. It isn't going to be easy. However if you succeed it will be worth it.

To offset my avoidance of fast food I grow my own vegetables. I like the exercise and I like the joy that is brought by gardening. I try and put a vegetable on every plate I eat. If you don't like the bitterness, look into ways that remove the bitter taste. You might be suffering from a bad memory brought on when you were a baby. An avoidance of vegetables could be from tasting it once and not liking it. Try to find a vegetable you do like the taste of. Don't be afraid.

• Calories

• Fat

• Nutrition Labels

• Vitamin A

• Food Deserts

• Eating Dessert

Chapter 5

How To Read A Nutrition Label

There is a method and a science to reading a nutrition label. It is important to ingest fat and calories. Salt is also important. You know those statins? Well, they are potentially life-saving and likely ordered by your doctor. Most statins cannot be ingested with grape fruit. Continue following your doctor's orders, but know that cholesterol levels aren't even a matter of study anymore. You know what they are studying? Phytochemicals and they are only found in plants.

I'm one of those people who obsessively read nutrition labels and I follow the rule that if I can't pronounce it, I don't eat it.

That's because I try and eat as wholesome as possible. I try to home cook all my meals and eat as many fruits and vegetables as possible. If you are someone who doesn't have time to cook, look into products that simplify the process.

Food really is medicine and everyone has to eat food every day. I was raised on agriculture. I know the in and outs of farm and farm living. Not everyone does, and everyone eats different.

Diet really isn't a one size fits all. There are simple rules that can guide you. Everything you eat should be done so in moderation. I eat several meals per day. I do eat breakfast and consider it the most important meal of the day. I pack in my protein and add extra if I am planning a big day at the gym. I love every bite of every burger I eat.

There is a lot to learn about nutrition and the reading of nutrition labels. If you want a simple formula know that your food should be as whole as possible. The average person should only get about 30 percent of their caloric intake from fats. Healthy fats from avocados and coconut oil are good. Fats from animals should be lessened. A plant-based diet is best. Beans are good. Everyone should have a colorful plate loaded with fruits and vegetables per day. Grains are not as important as some people have stated. Yes bread does taste good. It is not a necessary food. That includes all bread. Foods like blueberries and kale are considered superfoods. Nutrition does come with complications. The main problem is that so many companies make money trying to sell you diet advice. There is a nutritional science and there is a lot to learn about food. If you can't pronounce it, don't eat it. Try to buy as local as you can. Try to grow some of your own food. Food can do amazing things for you. Food was meant to be a healthy resource for us, not a controlling object. Everyone has to eat. You are killing things just by living. It is a life system that you are a part of. Life is a circle and healthy eating is a part of that circle. We are all animals and we need to feed ourselves as our bodies intended.

In many places in the country of the USA, the cooking is done in the basement. That is where people who love to cook really get down and do the nitty gritty work.

We've compiled a list for your ease.

· Nutrition Labels Are Intentionally Complicated

When you are reading a nutrition label and getting frustrated, know you are not alone. We recommend eating a whole-food diet rich in plants. If you can't pronounce it, you probably shouldn't eat it. Fats from calories should only be ingested at about 30 percent.

· Fats Are Good

Replace animal fats with healthy fats. Eat things like avocados and things made from coconut. Avoid margarines and transfats. Nuts are also a good source of protein.

· Supplements Are Good, But Don't Replace A Healthy Diet

There's no magic pill. If you don't like eating vegetables, consider trying to find a vegetable you do like to eat. Some vegetables I wrap in bacon in order to make them taste good.

· Eat Slow, Cook Slow

Avoid processed food and food with empty calories. Avoid soda. Eat everything in moderation. Don't eat too much of any one thing.

·Eat Healthy Fats

Foods like coconuts and avocados are rich in nutrients and have the good kind of fat your body craves.

Chapter 6

Money and Food

You can make a lot of money selling food. Think about it: everyone eats every day. In order to tell a part the charlatans those who really want to serve you healthy food, you have to know to get food from. The farm area I grew up in had a school shooting and in came all kinds of people trying to make money off of grief. I'll always remember how someone tried to sell someone a therapy pig. Well, if there's anything people in this area knows, is to tell the difference between a pig and a special pig. It was just a pig. The same thing goes with food. Avoid processed food and keep it as whole and close to nature as possible.

Think about spending a day at a farmers market and simply talking to the person who grows your food. This is a wonderful place you can network and get acquainted with locals. It's also a wonderful place to get closer to your food and your food place. Know where your food comes from.

Stick to your system and set yourself up for success. Let your system be your guide. You can be the manager of your plate. Did you know that cooking burns calories? Think about all the extra moving you will be doing cooking your own food. How much exactly does eating out cost you. Yes, the food tastes better and you don't have to do the dishes afterwards. It will drastically reduce your monthly grocery bill making your own food.

When you are in the dumps of life, you can rely on your system. Knowing you have responsibilities will help you through the tough times. Experts say that doing a simple task of eating breakfast every day can help. It is important to have individual tasks in order to maintain your health.

You also need to consider how important healthy food is to your family.

Food preparation really is a science and if you haven't taken a class of food born illnesses you should consider it. If you lose your way forgive yourself. Write down your system do that you can try it again. It's okay to fail as long as you pick yourself back up. That is the nature of food. If you take anything at all from this work, take away that there will be times of pain. It really is up to you to take that pain and turn it into something sweet that makes the world really see how wonderful life truly is. That's how nutrition really works. It really gives a glimpse into the reality of the human condition. Not everyone will have a big and immaculate kitchen and a refrigerator full of food. However, we all have value and there is a method to cooking without going crazy. With practice, anyone can become a home cook.

If you really want to be a cooking legend, then you need to know how to win. This book will help you navigate the world of nutrition.

Conclusion

Thank you again for downloading this book!

I hope this book was able to help you to clean your house.

The next step is to get working on your vehicle.

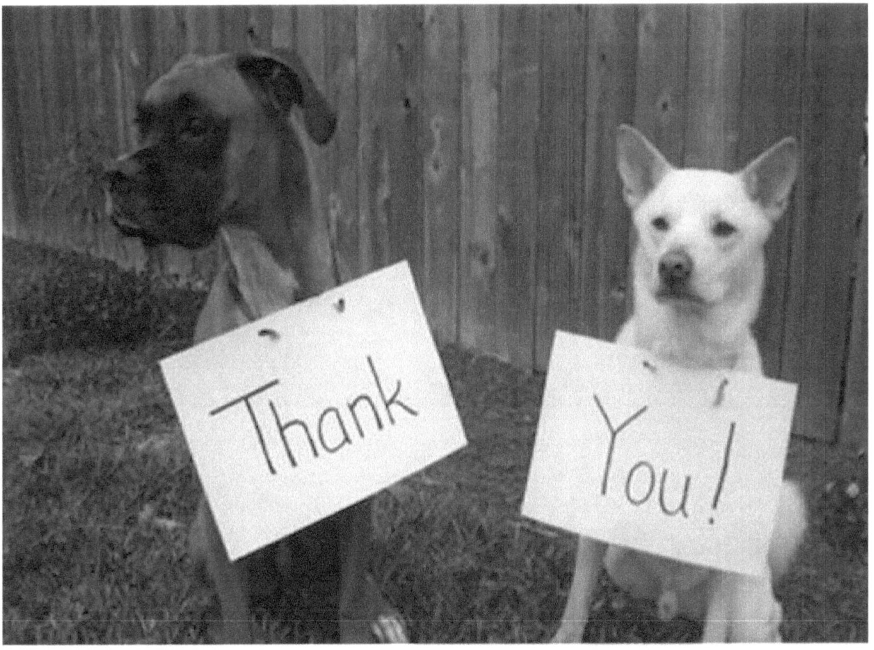

Finally, if you enjoyed this book, then I'd like to ask you for a favor, would you be kind enough to leave a review for this book on Amazon? It'd be greatly appreciated!

Thank you and good luck!

www.ingramcontent.com/pod-product-compliance
Lightning Source LLC
Chambersburg PA
CBHW051140250726
48655CB00007B/3158